**The Menopause Diet: 101
Main Dish, Breakf**
for Better Health and Natural Weight Loss

by **Alissa Noel Grey**
Text copyright(c)2015 Alissa Noel Grey

All rights reserved. No part of this publication may be reproduced, distributed, or transmitted in any form or by any means, including photocopying, recording, or other electronic or mechanical methods, without the prior written permission of the publisher, except in the case of brief quotations embodied in critical reviews and certain other noncommercial uses permitted by copyright law

Although every precaution has been taken to verify the accuracy of the information contained herein, the author and publisher assume no responsibility for any errors or omissions. No liability is assumed for damages that may result from the use of information contained within.

Table Of Contents

Living With the Menopause	6
Managing Menopause Symptoms Through Diet	7
Salad Recipes	10
Walnut Pesto Chicken Salad	11
Chicken, Broccoli and Tofu Salad	12
Turkey Quinoa Salad	13
Tuna and Green Bean Salad	14
Tuna Salad with Lettuce and Chickpeas	15
Bean and Tuna Salad	16
Beetroot and Carrot Salad with Salmon and Egg	17
Salmon and Quinoa Salad Recipe	18
Salmon and Avocado Salad	19
Spinach, Beet and Feta Salad	20
Summer Green Bean and Tofu Salad	21
Three Bean Salad	23
Beet and Bean Sprout Salad	25
Beet Salad with Walnuts	26
Warm Beet and Lentil Salad	27
Fried Zucchinis with Yogurt Sauce	28
Greek Cucumber and Yogurt Salad	29
Easy Artichoke and Bean Salad	30
Easy Vitamin Salad	31
Rainbow Superfood Salad	32
Shredded Kale and Brussels Sprout Salad	33
Quinoa and Zucchini Ribbon Salad	34
Quinoa and Avocado Salad	35
Fresh Quinoa Salad	36
Healthy Winter Quinoa Salad	37
Quinoa, Black Bean and Egg Salad	38
Quinoa, Kale and Roasted Pumpkin	39
Quinoa and Brussels Sprouts Salad	41
Easy Chickpea Salad	42
Homemade Hummus	43
Soup Recipes	44
Mediterranean Chicken Soup	45
Chicken and Butternut Squash Soup	46

Nettle Soup	47
Easy Fish Soup	48
Spanish Cold Prawn Soup	50
Leek, Brown Rice and Potato Soup	51
Easy Vegetable Soup	52
Curried Parsnip Soup	53
Mediterranean Chickpea Soup	54
Carrot, Sweet Potato and Chickpea Soup	55
Creamy Red Lentil Soup	56
Creamy Broccoli and Potato Soup	57
Creamy Brussels Sprouts Soup	58
Creamy Potato Soup	59
Lentil, Barley and Kale Soup	60
Mediterranean Lentil Soup	61
Pea, Dill and Brown Rice Soup	63
Minted Pea and Nettle Soup	64
Bean and Spinach Soup	65
Mushroom and Kale Soup	66
Quinoa, Sweet Potato and Tomato Soup	67
Red Lentil and Quinoa Soup	69
Spinach and Quinoa Soup	70
Vegetable Quinoa Soup	71
Kale, Leek and Quinoa Soup	72
Main Dish Recipes	73
Chicken and Zucchini Frittata	74
Hearty Chicken Spinach Frittata	75
Chicken and Mushroom Frittata	77
Greek Style Chicken Skewers	78
Chicken Puttanesca	79
Spinach with Ground Beef and Tofu	81
Ground Beef and Lentil Casserole	82
Salmon Kebabs	84
Mediterranean Baked Salmon	85
Simple Oven-Baked Sea Bass	86
Potato, Pea and Cauliflower Curry	87
Cauliflower with Chilli and Mustard	89
Baked Cauliflower	90
Maple Roast Parsnip with Pear and Sage	91

Balsamic Roasted Carrots and Baby Onions	92
Potato and Zucchini Bake	93
Creamy Avocado and Chicken Spaghetti	94
Easy Summer Spaghetti	95
One-pot Lentil and Olive Pasta	96
Summer Zucchini and Tofu Risotto	97
Vegetable Quinoa Stew	98
Eggplant and Qinoa Stew	99
Comforting Quinoa Shepherd's Stew	100
Easy Moroccan Vegetable Stew with Quinoa	102
Zucchini and Buckwheat Stew	104
Power Buckwheat Stew	105
Quick Buckwheat Chilli	106
Spicy Chickpea, Tofu and Spinach Stew	107
Moroccan Chickpea Stew	108
Chickpea, Rice and Mushroom Stew	110
Easy Chickpea Dinner	111
Baked Beans and Rice Casserole	112
Green Peas and Rice Casserole	113
Green Beans and Potatoes	114
Delicious Mushroom Tofu Pizza	115
Breakfast and Dessert Recipes	117
Avocado and Feta Toast with Poached Eggs	118
Avocado and Olive Paste on Toasted Rye Bread	119
Avocado, Lettuce and Tomato Sandwiches	120
Avocado and Chickpea Sandwiches	121
Quick Tofu and Vegetable Scramble	122
Raisin Quinoa Breakfast	123
Banana Cinnamon Fritters	124
Avocado and Banana Muffins	125
Avocado and Pumpkin Muffins	126
Oatmeal Muffins	127
Baked Apples	129
How To Lose Weight (During and) After Menopause?	130
FREE BONUS RECIPES: 20 Superfood Paleo and Vegan Smoothies for Vibrant Health and Easy Weight Loss	131
Kale and Kiwi Smoothie	132
Delicious Broccoli Smoothie	133

Papaya Smoothie	134
Beet and Papaya Smoothie	135
Lean Green Smoothie	136
Easy Antioxidant Smoothie	137
Healthy Purple Smoothie	138
Mom's Favorite Kale Smoothie	139
Creamy Green Smoothie	140
Strawberry and Arugula Smoothie	141
Emma's Amazing Smoothie	142
Good-To-Go Morning Smoothie	143
Endless Energy Smoothie	144
High-fibre Fruit Smoothie	145
Nutritious Green Smoothie	146
Apricot, Strawberry and Banana Smoothie	147
Spinach and Green Apple Smoothie	148
Superfood Blueberry Smoothie	149
Zucchini and Blueberry Smoothie	150
Tropical Spinach Smoothie	151
About the Author	152

Living With the Menopause

The menopause is a natural part of a woman's life, but it is also a signal that our bodies are changing. While it affects every woman differently, there is something that we all share – the menopause is a difficult time in our lives and we feel emotionally and physically on edge. The symptoms of the menopause vary considerably from one person to the next, but it is undeniable that the biological and psychological changes we all have to go through are not pleasant nor are they easy to ignore.

We know that menopause affects our energy levels, mood, sex drive, and memory, as well as our heart and bones. But there is another, equally distressing, symptom of this difficult time in a woman's life - changes in digestion. When estrogen levels drop and the effect of progesterone becomes more dominant we experience indigestion, heartburn, bloating, gas, constipation, and even gallstones. We also gain weight, especially around our bellies, and have difficulty losing it.

The good news is there are many things we can do to ensure that the menopause can be embraced rather than dreaded. Eating certain foods and avoiding others can reduce some of the symptoms and make the menopause a lot more bearable.

It is increasingly being found that good nutrition combined with small lifestyle changes can make a real difference to how we feel during our menopause. Good nutrition can also help us maintain a healthy weight and although there is no strict diet that we need to follow, it's particularly important that we have a balanced healthy diet, and regular meals, as irregular eating can make certain symptoms worse. And the earlier we make these important dietary changes, the easier the menopause and our life after the menopause is likely to be.

Managing Menopause Symptoms Through Diet

The basic principles of the menopause diet are relevant for anyone who wants to live a healthy life and lose weight, but are particularly suitable for women who are trying to get rid of the fat around their belly and reduce the hot flushes, and who want to enjoy life more.

1. Get More Phytoestrogens

Phytoestrogens are naturally-occurring plant nutrients that exert an estrogen-like action on the body. A high intake of phytoestrogens is thought to explain why hot flushes and other menopausal symptoms rarely occur in populations consuming a predominantly plant-based diet. We can increase our intake of phytoestrogens by eating more lentils, flaxseed, soy bean sprouts and soy milk, tofu, tempeh and miso, pumpkin seeds, sesame seeds, sunflower seeds, celery, rhubarb and green beans.

2. Eat More Fruit and Vegetables

- Fruit and vegetables are high in fiber, vitamins, minerals and antioxidants, and are naturally low in fat. They help us feel fuller longer, curb our appetite and control cravings.
- Eating a plant-based diet helps us maintain healthy cholesterol balance, prevents constipation and hence re-absorption of toxins to the body that are one of the reasons why we feel sluggish.
- Fruit and vegetables are a natural source of phytoestrogens that are very similar in structure to estrogen and act in a similar way. Adding phytoestrogen rich fruit and vegetables to our diet helps us keep hormones in balance and reduce hot flushes.
- Fruit and vegetables are delicious and healthy alternatives to sugary snacks and prevent a sharp rise in our blood sugar levels, followed by a sharp dip which leaves us feeling exhausted.
- The mineral boron is another very good reason we must

eat a predominantly plant based diet. Several studies have found evidence that consuming fruit and vegetables that contain boron increases the body's ability to hold onto estrogen and also helps our bones strength by decreasing the amount of calcium we lose each day and thus helps to reduce the risk of osteoporosis. Apples, pears, grapes, dates, raisins, legumes and nuts are good sources of boron.

3. Eat Fiber-rich Legumes

Beans, lentils, peas and chickpeas are good for women during and after the menopause because they are full of fiber, can slow the absorption of glucose in the bloodstream and curb our appetite. Legumes are also an amazing low-fat source of protein, contain phytoestrogens and are rich in vitamins and minerals, including calcium, folic acid and vitamin B-6.

4. Eat More of the Right Fats

- Always choose heart-healthy unsaturated fats such as olive and canola oil and try to consume more oils from nuts, seeds, and avocados.
- Eat more cold water fish such as salmon, tuna, herring, mackerel and halibut and eat less animal fat by choosing leaner meats and lower-fat dairy products.
- Avoid foods that contain hydrogenated and partially hydrogenated oils such as packaged cookies, chips, and crackers.

5. Get Adequate Calcium

Bone loss is a serious problem once hormone levels drop after the menopause and calcium is essential to our health as we age. To protect our bones' strength we need at least 1,000 mg of calcium daily from the age of 51 to 70. Sardines, salmon, broccoli, beans, kale, low-fat dairy, cottage or feta cheese, or even orange juice fortified with calcium can help us meet our calcium needs. To ensure that it is fully absorbed and deposited in our bones, it is best combined with foods rich in phosphorus such as peanuts, lean meat, cheese, onions, garlic and combined with vitamin D which is found in oily fish, lentils, eggs and brown rice.

6. Eat Complex Carbohydrates

Always choose complex carbohydrates over refined carbohydrates such as white bread, white pasta, cakes, etc. Foods such as quinoa, buckwheat, potatoes, whole-wheat pasta, brown rice and oatmeal boost our feel-good serotonin levels without causing an energy crash. Foods that provide complex carbohydrates are also rich in fiber, so we feel full much longer and don't experience the dip which leaves us feeling tired and drained.

7. Boost Energy with High-quality Lean Protein

As we enter the menopausal years, we start to lose muscle, strength and bone mass at a greater rate. Including mostly lean sources of protein in our diet helps control our calorie and saturated fat intake, makes us feel full longer and, most importantly, helps us preserve lean body mass. Fish, cottage cheese, nuts, beans, eggs and quinoa are lean, nutrient-rich, protein-packed dietary staples that we need to include in our everyday menu in order to be healthy and diminish menopausal symptoms.

Salad Recipes

Walnut Pesto Chicken Salad

Serves: 4

Prep time: 10 min

Ingredients:

2 cups cooked chicken, diced

1 large apple, peeled and diced

1 large avocado, peeled and diced

for the walnut pesto

1/2 cup walnuts, chopped

10 fresh basil leaves

1 garlic clove

2-3 green olives

4 tbsps extra virgin olive oil

1 tbsp lemon juice

salt and black pepper, to taste

Directions:

In a food processor, blend together walnuts, olives, basil, olive oil, garlic and lemon juice until completely smooth.

Combine diced chicken, apple, and avocado. Pour over the walnut pesto, stir to combine and serve.

Chicken, Broccoli and Tofu Salad

Serves: 4

Prep time: 5-6 min

Ingredients:

2 lbs broccoli, cut into florets

4 oz firm tofu

1/2 cup red onion, chopped

1 cup cooked chicken breasts, diced

1 cup mozzarella cheese, grated

1/2 cup fresh parsley leaves, finely cut

2 tbsp extra virgin olive oil

2 tbsp soy sauce

2 tbsp lemon juice

Directions:

Steam broccoli for 4-5 minutes until just tender. Mix it with the chicken pieces.

Wrap tofu with fine cotton cloth and squeeze out to remove some water. Crumble it tofu and add it to the broccoli. Add in onion and finely cut parsley and combine very well.

In a smaller cup, mix the olive oil, soy sauce and lemon juice. Pour over the salad, toss to combine and serve.

Turkey Quinoa Salad

Serves: 4

Prep time: 10 min

Ingredients:

1/2 cup quinoa

1 cup water

1 cup skinless lean turkey breast, cooked, diced

1/2 red onion, chopped

1/2 cup dried cranberries

1/2 cup walnuts

1 cup soy bean sprouts

2 tbsp extra virgin olive oil

1 tbsp lemon juice

salt and black pepper, to taste

Directions:

Wash quinoa with lots of water and boil it according to package directions.

Set aside in a salad bowl and fluff with a fork. Add in turkey, onion, cranberries and walnuts and toss to combine.

Whisk olive oil, lemon juice, salt and pepper in a separate bowl and pour over the salad. Sprinkle with soy bean sprouts, toss again, and serve.

Tuna and Green Bean Salad

Serves: 4

Prep time: 5 min

Ingredients:

12 oz mixed greens, washed and dried

9 oz green beans, trimmed and cut into 2-inch length

1 cup cherry tomatoes, halved

1 ripe avocado, peeled and sliced

1 cup black olives, pitted, halved

1 can tuna, drained and broken into chunks

3 tbsp extra virgin olive oil

2 tbsp lemon juice

2 tbsp Dijon mustard

Directions:

Cook the green beans in boiling water for 3-4 minutes. Drain and set aside to cool.

Prepare the dressing by combining together olive oil, lemon juice and mustard. Season with salt and black pepper to taste.

Combine the beans, mixed greens, cherry tomatoes, avocado, tuna, and the dressing. Toss gently and serve.

Tuna Salad with Lettuce and Chickpeas

Serves: 4

Prep time: 5 min

Ingredients:

1 head green lettuce, washed cut in thin strips

1 cup chopped watercress

1 cucumber, peeled and chopped

1 tomato, diced

1 can tuna, drained and broken into small chunks

1/2 cup chickpeas, from a can

10 radishes, sliced

3-4 spring onions, chopped

juice of half lemon

3 tbsp extra virgin olive oil

2 tbsp raw pumpkin seeds

Directions:

Mix all the vegetables in a large bowl. Add the tuna and the chickpeas and season with lemon juice, oil and salt to taste.

Sprinkle with pumpkin seeds and serve.

Bean and Tuna Salad

Serves: 4

Prep time: 5 min

Ingredients:

1 can white beans, rinsed and drained

1 cup canned tuna, drained and broken into chunks

1 small red onion, chopped

1 avocado, peeled and sliced or chopped

juice of one lemon

1/2 cup fresh parsley leaves, chopped

1 tsp dried mint

salt and black pepper, to taste

3 tbsp extra virgin olive oil

Directions:

Put tuna chunks and beans in a salad bowl and toss to combine. Add in avocado, onions, parsley, mint, lemon juice and olive oil and mix to combine.

Season with salt and black pepper to taste. Serve chilled.

Beetroot and Carrot Salad with Salmon and Egg

Serves: 4

Prep time: 10 min

Ingredients:

2 eggs, hardboiled and crushed

1 beet, peeled and grated

3 carrots, peeled and grated

4 oz smoked salmon, flaked

1 small red onion, chopped

1/4 cup fresh lemon juice

2 tbsp extra virgin olive oil

salt and black pepper, to taste

Directions:

In a large bowl, gently toss together the salmon, onion, carrots, beet, and crushed hard-boiled eggs.

Prepare the dressing by whisking lemon juice and olive oil in a small bowl. Season with salt and pepper and drizzle over over the salad.

Salmon and Quinoa Salad Recipe

Serves: 4

Prep time: 20 min

Ingredients:

1/2 cup quinoa

1 cups water

2 cups cooked and flaked salmon

1/2 red bell pepper, chopped

1/2 cup canned beans, drained

1 tsp Dijon mustard

1 tsp lemon juice

5-6 spring onions, chopped

3 tbsp fresh parsley leaves, finely cut

freshly ground black pepper, to taste

Directions:

Rinse quinoa in a fine sieve under cold running water and boil it in one cup of water for 15 minutes. Fluff with a fork and set aside.

In a large salad bowl, mix the salmon, red bell pepper, spring onions, parsley, mustard and lemon juice. Stir in the cooked quinoa.

Season with freshly ground black pepper to taste and toss to combine. Serve chilled.

Salmon and Avocado Salad

Serves 4

Prep time: 5 min

Ingredients:

2 cups cooked, flaked salmon

1 cucumber, peeled and diced

1 avocado, peeled and cubed

1 cup soy bean sprouts, trimmed

4-5 radishes, sliced

4 to 5 tbsp mayonnaise, or enough to moisten

1 tbsp lemon juice

1 tbsp dill, very finely chopped

Directions:

Place cucumber, avocado, soy bean sprouts, radishes and salmon into a salad bowl and toss well to combine.

Add in mayonnaise, season with salt and pepper to taste, sprinkle with dill and lemon juice, and serve.

Spinach, Beet and Feta Salad

Serves: 4-5

Prep time: 15 min

Ingredients:

3 medium beets, steamed, peeled and diced

1 bag baby spinach leaves

1/2 cup walnuts, toasted

4 oz feta, crumbled

4-5 spring onions, chopped

for the dressing:

1 garlic clove, crushed

2 tbsp extra virgin olive oil

2 tbsp lemon juice

1 tbsp finely chopped dill

Directions:

Wash the beets well, steam, peel and dice them. Arrange the spinach leaves in a large salad bowl. Scatter the beets, onions, walnuts and feta over the spinach.

In a smaller bowl or cup, combine the oil, lemon juice, garlic and dill. Whisk until smooth, season with salt and pepper, and drizzle over the salad.

Summer Green Bean and Tofu Salad

Serves: 4

Prep time: 10 min

Ingredients:

1 lb trimmed green beans, cut into 2-inch long pieces

1 small red onion, finely cut

1 cup cherry tomatoes, halved

1 avocado, peeled, pitted and cut

3-4 garlic cloves, chopped

10 oz extra-firm tofu, cubed

2 tbsp peanut oil

4 tbsp extra virgin olive oil

3/4 cup freshly grated Parmesan cheese

salt and pepper, to taste

Directions:

Steam or boil the green beans for about 3-4 minutes until crisp-tender. In a colander, wash with cold water to stop cooking, then pat dry and place in a salad bowl.

Slice the tofu into quarters, press to remove excess moisture and cut into cubes. Heat a cast iron pan over medium-high heat, then add peanut oil and add the tofu in a single layer. Sprinkle it with salt and black pepper to taste and brown on all sides. Add to the green beans.

Stir in red onion, garlic, cherry tomatoes and avocado, season with lemon juice and balsamic vinegar and toss to coat.

Sprinkle in the olive oil and Parmesan cheese and toss again. Season to taste with salt and freshly ground black pepper and serve.

Three Bean Salad

Serves: 4

Prep time: 15 min

Ingredients:

½ cup canned chickpeas, drained and rinsed

½ cup canned kidney beans, drained and rinsed

1 lb trimmed green beans, cut into 2-3 inch long pieces

a bunch of radishes, sliced

5-6 green onions, chopped

½ cup cilantro leaves, finely cut

for the dressing:

2 tbsp honey

½ tsp ground dry mustard

1 tsp garlic powder

3 tbsp extra virgin olive oil

4 tbsp apple cider vinegar

1/4 tsp ground black pepper

Directions:

Steam or boil the green beans for about 3-4 minutes until crisp-tender. In a colander, wash with cold water to stop cooking, pat dry and place in a salad bowl.

Add in the chickpeas, kidney beans, green onions, radishes and cilantro leaves.

In a smaller bowl, whisk together the apple cider vinegar, olive oil, honey, mustard, garlic powder, black pepper and salt. Pour over the salad and toss gently to coat. Cover, refrigerate for at least 1 hour, toss again and serve.

Beet and Bean Sprout Salad

Serves: 4

Prep time: 10 min

Ingredients:

5-6 beet greens, finely cut

2 tomatoes, sliced

1 cup bean sprouts, washed

1/2 cup pine nuts

for the dressing:

2 garlic cloves, crushed

4 tbsp lemon juice

4 tbsp extra virgin olive oil

1 tsp salt

Directions:

Place the pine nuts in a small pan over medium heat and cook for 2 minutes, stirring regularly, or until golden. Remove from heat and set aside.

In a large salad bowl, toss together beet greens, bean sprouts and tomatoes.

Whisk the olive oil, lemon juice, salt and garlic together and pour the mixture over the salad. Sprinkle with pine nuts and serve chilled.

Beet Salad with Walnuts

Serves: 4

Prep time: 15 min

Ingredients:

3 medium beets, steamed and diced

1 red onion, sliced

1/2 cup walnuts, halved

1 tbsp lemon juice

2 tbsp olive oil

4-5 mint leaves

½ tsp salt

Directions:

Wash the beets, trim the stems, and steam them over boiling water until cooked through. When they are cool enough to handle, peel and dice them.

Place the beets in a salad bowl, add in walnuts, onion, lemon juice and olive oil and toss to combine.

Refrigerate and serve sprinkled with fresh mint leaves.

Warm Beet and Lentil Salad

Serves: 5-6

Prep time: 10 min

Ingredients:

1 14 oz can brown lentils, drained, rinsed

1 14 oz can sliced pickled beets, drained

1 cup baby arugula leaves

1 small red onion, chopped

2 garlic cloves, crushed

6 oz feta cheese, crumbled

1 tbsp extra virgin olive oil

for the dressing

3 tbsp extra virgin olive oil

1 tbsp red wine vinegar

1 tsp summer savory

salt and black pepper, to taste

Directions:

Heat one tablespoon of olive oil in a frying pan and gently sauté onion for 2-3 minutes or until softened. Add in garlic, lentils and beets. Cook, stirring, for 2 minutes.

Whisk together remaining olive oil, vinegar, summer savory, salt and pepper. Add to the lentils and toss to coat. Combine baby arugula, feta and lentil mixture in a bowl. Toss gently to combine and serve.

Fried Zucchinis with Yogurt Sauce

Serves: 4

Prep time: 20 min

Ingredients:

4 medium-sized zucchinis, peeled and cut into 1/4-inch thick slices

1 ½ cup Greek yogurt

3 cloves garlic, crushed

1 cup chopped fresh dill

1 cup all-purpose flour

2 cups sunflower oil

2 tbsp flaxseed

salt, to taste

Directions:

Combining the garlic and chopped dill with the yogurt and flaxseed in a small bowl. Add salt to taste and set aside.

Wash and dry zucchinis, and cut into 1/4-inch thick slices. Salt and leave them in a strainer to drain away the juices.

Coat the zucchinis with flour, then fry in sunflower oil, turning on both sides until they are golden-brown (about 3 minutes on each side). Transfer to paper towels and pat dry. Serve old, with garlic yogurt on the side.

Greek Cucumber and Yogurt Salad

Serves: 5-6

Prep time: 10 min

Ingredients:

2 large cucumbers, peeled and finely chopped

3 cups Greek yogurt

1/3 cup crushed walnuts

2-3 cloves garlic, crushed

1/2 cup chopped fresh mint

1 tbsp flaxseed

2 tbsp extra virgin olive oil

salt, to taste

Directions:

Strain the yogurt in a piece of cheesecloth or a clean white dishtowel.

Put the finely chopped cucumbers in a sieve and press out as much excess liquid as possible. Place them in a deep bowl and add in the walnuts, the flaxseed and the crushed garlic, the oil and the finely chopped mint. Scoop the drained yogurt into the bowl and stir well.

Season with salt to the taste and put in the fridge for at least an hour.

Easy Artichoke and Bean Salad

Serves: 5-6

Prep time: 15 min

Ingredients:

1 14 oz can white beans, drained

2-3 large handfuls podded broad beans

3 marinated artichoke hearts, quartered

for the dressing:

2 tbsp extra virgin olive oil

1 tbsp lemon juice

1 tbsp apple cider vinegar

1 tbsp fresh mint, chopped

salt and pepper, to taste

Directions:

Cook the broad beans in boiling, unsalted water for 2-3 minutes or until tender. Drain and refresh under running cold water. Combine with the white beans and quartered marinated artichoke hearts in a large salad bowl.

In a smaller bowl, whisk olive oil, lemon juice, vinegar and mint. Pour over the bean mixture. Season with salt and pepper and toss gently to combine.

Easy Vitamin Salad

Serves: 4-5

Prep time: 10 min

Ingredients:

6 small new potatoes

1 carrot, peeled and cut

7 oz cauliflower, cut into florets

7 oz baby Brussels sprouts, trimmed

3-4 broccoli florets

for the dressing:

3 tbsp fresh lemon juice

2 tbsp extra virgin olive oil

2 garlic cloves, crushed

Directions:

Cook potatoes in a steamer basket over boiling water for 10 minutes or until just tender. Add in the cauliflower, broccoli and Brussels sprouts and cook for 5 minutes more.

Using a vegetable peeler, cut thin ribbons from carrot. Add to the steam basket and cook for 4 minutes more. Refresh under cold running water and set aside for to cool.

Whisk the lemon juice, oil, and garlic in a small bowl. Season with salt and pepper.

Cut the potatoes in half lengthways and place them in a salad bowl. Add in cauliflower, Brussels sprouts, carrot and broccoli. Pour the dressing over the salad and gently toss to combine.

Rainbow Superfood Salad

Serves: 4-5

Prep time: 10 min

Ingredients:

2 cups shredded red cabbage

1 cup broccoli or sunflower sprouts

1 medium cucumber

1 red apple

1 carrot, peeled

for the dressing:

1 tbsp red wine vinegar

2 tbsp extra virgin olive oil

1 tsp sumac

salt and pepper, to taste

Directions:

Using a vegetable peeler, cut thin ribbons from carrot, cucumber and apple. Place in a large bowl. Add cabbage and sprouts.

Whisk ingredients for the dressing until smooth. Pour over salad, toss to combine and serve.

Shredded Kale and Brussels Sprout Salad

Serves: 4-6

Prep time: 20 min

Ingredients:

18-29 Brussels sprouts, shredded

1 cup finely shredded kale

1/2 cup grated Parmesan or Pecorino cheese

1 cup walnuts, halved, toasted

1/2 cup dried cranberries

for the dressing:

6 tbsp extra virgin olive oil

2 tbsp apple cinder vinegar

1 tbsp Dijon mustard

salt and pepper, to taste

Directions:

Shred the Brussels sprouts and kale in a food processor or mandolin. Toss them in a bowl, top with toasted walnuts, cranberries and grated cheese.

In a smaller bowl, whisk the olive oil, apple cider vinegar and mustard until smooth. Pour the dressing over the salad, stir and serve.

Quinoa and Zucchini Ribbon Salad

Serves: 4

Prep time: 15 min

Ingredients:

1 cup quinoa

2 cups water

1 zucchini, sliced lengthwise into thin ribbons (a mandoline is ideal)

3-4 green onions, chopped

1 cup cherry tomatoes, halved

4 oz feta, crumbled or cut in small cubes

2 tbsp extra virgin olive oil

3 tbsp lemon juice

salt, to taste

Directions:

Heat oil in a large saucepan over medium-high heat. Add zucchini and and cook, stirring, until zucchini is crisp-tender, about 4 minutes. Set aside in a plate.

Wash quinoa in a fine mesh strainer under running water for 1-2 minutes, then set aside to drain. Bring water to a boil in a medium saucepan over high heat. Add in the quinoa and return to a boil. Cover, reduce heat to a simmer and cook gently for 15 minutes. Set aside, covered, for 5-6 minutes.

Toss quinoa with zucchini, green onions, tomatoes, lemon juice and olive oil. Serve warm or room temperature, topped with feta cheese.

Quinoa and Avocado Salad

Serves: 4

Prep time: 15 min

Ingredients:

1 cup quinoa

2 cups water

1 large avocado, pitted and sliced

¼ radicchio, finely sliced

1 small pink grapefruit, peeled and finely cut

1 handful arugula

1 cup baby spinach leaves

2 tbsp extra virgin olive oil

2 tbsp lemon juice

salt and black pepper, to taste

Directions:

Wash quinoa in a fine sieve under running water for 2-3 minutes, or until water runs clear. Set aside to drain, then boil it in two cups of water for 15 minutes.

Fluff with a fork and set aside to cool. Stir avocado, radicchio, arugula and baby spinach into cooled quinoa. Add grapefruit, lemon juice, and olive oil, season with salt and black pepper and stir to combine well.

Fresh Quinoa Salad

Serves: 4-5

Prep time: 15 min

Ingredients:

1 cup quinoa, rinsed

2 cups water

1 large cucumber, diced

1 big tomato, diced

1 yellow pepper, chopped

6-7 arugula leaves

½ cup fresh dill, finely cut

for the dressing:

3 tbsp lemon juice

3 tbsp extra virgin olive oil

salt and black pepper, to taste

Directions:

Wash quinoa in a fine mesh strainer under running water for 1-2 minutes, then set aside to drain. Bring water to a boil in a medium saucepan over high heat. Add the quinoa and return to a boil.

Cover, reduce heat to a simmer and cook gently for 15 minutes. Set aside, covered, for 5-6 minutes, then transfer to a large bowl and mix with the cucumber, tomato, pepper, arugula and dill.

I a small bowl, combine the lemon juice, olive oil, salt and black pepper. Pour over the salad and toss to combine.

Healthy Winter Quinoa Salad

Serves: 4

Prep time: 20 min

Ingredients:

½ cup quinoa

1 cup water

1-2 small beets, peeled, boiled and grated

1 apple, peeled and shredded

2 oz crumbled feta

3-4 green onions, finely cut

½ bunch of fresh parsley, finely cut

2 tbsp lemon juice

1 tsp chia seeds

3 tbsp extra virgin olive oil

salt, to taste

Directions:

Wash quinoa in a fine sieve under running water for 2-3 minutes, or until water runs clear. Set aside to drain, then boil in a cup of water for 15 minutes.

Steam the beets in a basket over a pot of boiling water for about 12-15 minutes, or until tender. Leave them to cool then grate and put them in a salad bowl. Add the finely cut green onions, shredded apple, feta cheese and fresh parsley and mix well.

Season with salt, lemon juice and olive oil, add quinoa and chia and stir to combine well.

Quinoa, Black Bean and Egg Salad

Serves: 4-5

Prep time: 15 min

Ingredients:

1 cup quinoa

2 cups water

1 cup canned black beans, drained

1 tomato, sliced

2-3 green onions, chopped

2 eggs, hard boiled, peeled and sliced

½ cup fresh cilantro, finely cut

1 tsp dried mint

3 tbsp lemon juice

4 tbsp extra virgin olive oil

½ tsp salt

Directions:

Wash quinoa in a fine sieve under running water for 2-3 minutes, or until water runs clear. Set aside to drain, then boil in two cups of water for 15 minutes.

Put beans, tomato, green onions, eggs and cilantro in a bowl and toss with lemon juice, olive oil, dried mint and salt. Add in quinoa and toss to combine. Serve and Enjoy!

Quinoa, Kale and Roasted Pumpkin

Serves: 4-5

Prep time: 30-35 min

Ingredients:

1 cup quinoa

2 cups water

1.5 lb pumpkin, peeled and seeded, cut into cubes

2 cups fresh kale, chopped

5 oz crumbled feta cheese

1 large onion, finely chopped

4-5 tbsp extra virgin olive oil

1 tsp finely grated ginger

½ tsp cumin

½ tsp salt

Directions:

Preheat oven to 350 F. Line a baking tray and arrange the pumpkin cubes on on it. Drizzle with 2-3 tablespoons of olive oil and salt. Toss to coat, place in the oven and cook for 20-25 minutes, stirring every 10 minutes.

Heat the remaining olive oil in a large saucepan over medium-high heat. Gently sauté onion, for 2-3 minutes, or until softened. Add the spices and cook, stirring, for 1 minute more.

Wash quinoa under running water until the water runs clear. Bring two cups of water to a boil and add quinoa. Reduce heat to low, cover, and simmer for 15 minutes.

Stir in kale and cook until it wilts. Gently combine quinoa and kale mixture with the roasted pumpkin and sautéed onion.

Quinoa and Brussels Sprouts Salad

Serves: 5-6

Prep time: 20-25 min

Ingredients:

1 cup quinoa

2 cups water

4 cups Brussels sprouts, halved

2 leeks, washed, trimmed and sliced

½ cup walnuts, chopped

½ cup dried cranberries

½ cup fresh parsley, chopped

2 tbsp balsamic vinegar

3 tbsp extra virgin olive oil

Directions:

Preheat the oven to 350 F. Line a baking tray and arrange Brussels sprouts and leeks on it. Drizzle with olive oil, balsamic vinegar and salt and toss to coat. Roast about 20-25 minutes.

Wash quinoa under running water until the water runs clear. Bring two cups of water to a boil and add quinoa. Reduce heat to low, cover, and simmer for 10 minutes then fluff with a fork and set aside.

In a salad bowl, toss together the quinoa, roasted vegetables, walnuts and cranberries. Season with salt and pepper to taste and serve.

Easy Chickpea Salad

Serves: 3-4

Prep time: 2-3 min

Ingredients:

1 15 oz can chickpeas, drained

1 medium red onion, finely cut

1 cucumber, peeled and diced

2 tomatoes, sliced

a bunch of radishes, sliced

½ cup fresh parsley, finely chopped

2 tbsp extra virgin olive oil

1 tbsp balsamic vinegar

salt, to taste

4 oz crumbled feta cheese, to serve

Directions:

In a salad bowl, toss together the chickpeas, onion, cucumber, tomatoes, radishes and parsley.

Add in the balsamic vinegar, olive oil and salt and stir. Serve sprinkled with crumbled feta cheese.

Homemade Hummus

Serves: 5-6

Prep time: 5 min

Ingredients:

1 15 oz can chickpeas, drained

3-4 tbsp tahini paste

3 tbsp extra virgin olive oil

½ lemon, juiced

2-3 small garlic cloves, chopped, or to taste

1-2 tsp cumin, or to taste

1 tsp salt

water from the chickpea can

extra virgin olive oil, parsley, paprika for serving

Directions:

Drain the chickpeas and keep the juice in a small cup. If possible, remove the skins from the chickpeas. Place the chickpeas in a blender and pulse. Add the tahini, lemon juice, garlic, olive oil, cumin and salt and blend until smooth, gradually adding the chickpea water to the mix until the mixture is completely smooth.

To serve, top with olive oil, parsley, and sprinkle with paprika.

Soup Recipes

Mediterranean Chicken Soup

Serves: 4

Prep time: 35 min

Ingredients:

3 chicken breasts

1 carrot, chopped

1 small zucchini, peeled and chopped

1 celery stalk, chopped

1 small onion, chopped

1 cup canned chickpeas, drained

1 bay leaf

6 cups water

6-7 black olives, pitted and halved

1/2 tsp salt

black pepper, to taste

fresh parsley, to serve

lemon juice, to serve

Directions:

Place chicken breasts, onion, carrot, celery, chickpeas and bay leaf in a deep soup pot. Add in salt, black pepper and 6 cups of water. Stir well and bring to a boil. Add zucchini and olives and reduce heat. Simmer for 30 minutes.

Remove chicken from the pot and set aside to cool. Shred it and return it back to the pot. Serve with lemon juice and sprinkled with parsley.

Chicken and Butternut Squash Soup

Serves: 4

Prep time: 35 min

Ingredients:

3 boneless chicken thighs, diced

1/2 onion, chopped

6-7 white mushrooms chopped

1 small zucchini, peeled and diced

1 cup butternut squash, diced

1 tbsp tomato paste

5 cups water

1/4 tsp cumin

1 tbsp paprika

3 tbsp extra virgin olive oil

Directions:

In a deep soup pot, heat olive oil and gently sauté onion, stirring occasionally. Add chicken and cook for 2-3 minutes. Stir in cumin, paprika and butternut squash.

Dilute the tomato paste in a cup of water and add to the soup. Add in the remaining water and bring to a boil.

Reduce heat and simmer for 10 minutes then add zucchini and mushrooms. Simmer until butternut squash is tender. Season with salt and black pepper to taste.

Nettle Soup

Serves 6-7

Prep time: 20 min

Ingredients:

2 lbs young top shoots of nettles, well washed

2 potatoes, diced small

5-6 spring onions, chopped

3 cups water

1 cup soy milk

3-4 tbsp extra virgin olive oil

1 tsp salt

3 tbsp chopped fresh mint

Directions:

Clean the nettles, wash and cook them in slightly salted water for 1-2 minutes.

Discard the water and chop the nettles finely.

In a soup pot, gently sauté the spring onions and potatoes in olive oil for 2-3 minutes, stirring. Add in the nettles and 3 cups of water. Stir well, then simmer until the potatoes are cooked through.

Add soy milk, blend until smooth, sprinkle with mint and serve.

Easy Fish Soup

Serves 6-7

Prep time: 20 min

Ingredients:

1 lb white fish fillets cut in small pieces

1 onion, diced

1 celery stalk, chopped

2 tomatoes, chopped

3 potatoes, peeled and diced

1 red pepper, chopped

2 carrots, chopped

3 garlic cloves, crushed

1 bay leaf

3 tbsp extra virgin olive oil

1 chilli, seeded and crushed

1 tsp dried dill

½ tsp ground black pepper

4 cups water or fish stock

1 cup finely cut parsley

Directions:

Gently heat the olive oil over medium heat and sauté the onion, celery, red pepper, garlic and carrots until tender.

Stir in the chilli, bay leaf, salt, and pepper. Add in water, potatoes and tomatoes and bring to a boil.

Reduce heat, cover, and cook until the potatoes are almost done. Stir in the fish and cook until fish is easily flaked with fork, about 10 minutes. Stir in the parsley and serve hot.

Spanish Cold Prawn Soup

Serves 8-9

Prep time: 20 min

Ingredients:

3 lbs cooked, peeled and deveined prawn

3 cups tomato juice

3 cups prawn stock

3 spring onions, chopped

3 avocados, peeled and diced

1 cucumber, peeled and diced

2 large tomatoes, diced

1 cup finely chopped parsley

2 tbsp lime juice

salt and pepper, to taste

Directions:

Combine the tomato juice and prawn stock. Stir in the prawns, avocados, cucumber, tomatoes, spring onions, parsley, lime juice, salt and pepper.

Refrigerate until ready to serve.

Leek, Brown Rice and Potato Soup

Serves: 4-5

Prep time: 35 min

Ingredients:

3 potatoes, peeled and diced

2 leeks, finely chopped

1/4 cup brown rice

5 cups water

3 tbsp extra virgin olive oil

lemon juice, to taste

Directions:

Heat olive oil in a deep soup pot and sauté leeks for 3-4 minutes. Add in potatoes and cook for a minute more. Stir in water, bring to a boil, and the brown rice.

Reduce heat and simmer for 30 minutes. Add lemon juice, to taste, and serve.

Easy Vegetable Soup

Serves: 4-5

Prep time: 35 min

Ingredients:

2 leeks, white parts only, well rinsed and thinly sliced

1 carrot, chopped

1 cup Brussels sprouts, halved

1 potato, peeled and diced

1 garlic clove, chopped

1 red pepper, chopped

1 yellow pepper, chopped

1 cup white mushrooms, halved

4 cups vegetable broth

3 tbsp extra virgin olive oil

salt and black pepper, to taste

Directions:

Heat the olive oil in a large soup pot. Add in the leeks and cook over low heat for 2-3 minutes. Add in the Brussels sprouts, carrot, garlic, peppers and potato and cook for about 5 minutes, stirring. Add the vegetable broth and the mushrooms and bring to a boil.

Reduce heat and simmer, uncovered, for 30 minutes, or until the vegetables are tender but still holding their shape. Season with salt and pepper to taste and serve.

Curried Parsnip Soup

Serves: 4-5

Prep time: 40 min

Ingredients:

1.5 lb parsnips, peeled, chopped

1 onion, chopped

2 garlic cloves, chopped

4 cups water

2 tbsp extra virgin olive oil

1 tbs curry powder

1/2 cup soy milk

salt and black pepper, to taste

Directions:

In a deep saucepan, gently sauté the onion and garlic together with the curry powder. Add in the parsnips and sauté, stirring often, for 5-6 minutes. Add water, bring to a boil, and simmer for 30 minutes or until the parsnips are tender.

Set aside to cool then blend in batches until smooth. Return soup to the pan, stir in the soy milk and heat through. Season with salt and pepper to taste.

Mediterranean Chickpea Soup

Serves 4-5

Prep time: 30 min

Ingredients:

1 can (15 oz) chickpeas, drained

1 onion, chopped

2-3 garlic cloves, chopped

1 celery stalk, finely cut

1 can tomatoes, diced

2 cups water

2 cups soy milk

3 tbsp extra virgin olive oil

1-2 bay leaves

1/2 tsp dried oregano

Directions:

In a soup pot, heat olive oil and gently sauté onion, celery and garlic for 1-2 minutes. Add in water, chickpeas, tomatoes, bay leaves, and oregano.

Bring to a boil then reduce heat, and simmer for 20 minutes. Add in soy milk and cook for 1-2 minutes more. Set aside to cool, discard the bay leaves and blend until smooth.

Carrot, Sweet Potato and Chickpea Soup

Serves: 5-6

Prep time: 35 min

Ingredients:

3 large carrots, chopped

1/2 onion, chopped

1 can (15 oz) chickpeas, undrained

2 sweet potatoes, peeled and diced

4 cups vegetable broth

2 tbsp extra virgin olive oil

1 tsp cumin

1 tsp ginger

Directions:

Heat olive oil in a large saucepan over medium heat. Add onion and carrots and sauté until tender. Add in broth, chickpeas, sweet potato and seasonings.

Bring to a boil then reduce heat and simmer, covered, for 30 minutes. Blend soup until smooth, add in coconut milk and cook for 2-3 minutes until heated through.

Creamy Red Lentil Soup

Serves: 4-5

Prep time: 40 min

Ingredients:

1 cup red lentils

1/2 small onion, chopped

2 garlic cloves, chopped

1/2 red pepper, chopped

3 cups vegetable broth

1 cup coconut milk

3 tbsp extra virgin olive oil

1 tbsp paprika

1/2 tsp ginger

1 tsp cumin

salt and black pepper, to taste

Directions:

Gently heat olive oil in a large saucepan. Add onion, garlic, red pepper, paprika, ginger and cumin and sauté, stirring, until fragrant. Add in red lentils and vegetable broth.

Bring to a boil, cover, and simmer for 35 minutes. Add in coconut milk and simmer for 5 more minutes. Remove from heat, season with salt and black pepper, and blend until smooth. Serve hot.

Creamy Broccoli and Potato Soup

Serves: 4-5

Prep time: 30 min

Ingredients:

3 cups broccoli, chopped

2 potatoes, peeled and chopped

1 onion, chopped

3 garlic cloves, chopped

1 cup raw cashews

1 cup vegetable broth

4 cups water

3 tbsp extra virgin olive oil

1/2 tsp ground nutmeg

Directions:

Soak cashews in a bowl covered with water for at least 4 hours. Drain water and blend cashews with 1 cup of vegetable broth until smooth. Set aside.

Gently heat olive oil in a large saucepan over medium-high heat. Cook onion and garlic and for 3-4 minutes until tender. Add in broccoli, potato, nutmeg and water. Cover and bring to the boil, then reduce heat and simmer for 20 minutes, stirring from time to time.

Remove from heat and stir in cashew mixture. Blend until smooth, return to pan and cook until heated through.

Creamy Brussels Sprouts Soup

Serves: 4-5

Prep time: 30 min

Ingredients:

1 lb frozen Brussels sprouts, thawed

2 potatoes, peeled and chopped

1 large onion, chopped

3 garlic cloves, minced

1 cup raw cashews

4 cups vegetable broth

3 tbsp extra virgin olive oil

1/2 tsp curry powder

salt and black pepper, to taste

Directions:

Soak cashews in a bowl covered with water for at least 4 hours. Drain water and blend cashews with 1 cup of vegetable broth until smooth. Set aside.

Gently heat olive oil in a large saucepan over medium-high heat. Cook onion and garlic and for 3-4 minutes until tender. Add in Brussels sprouts, potato, curry and vegetable broth. Cover and bring to a boil, then reduce heat and simmer for 20 minutes, stirring from time to time.

Remove from heat and stir in cashew mixture. Blend until smooth, return to pan and cook until heated through.

Creamy Potato Soup

Serves: 4-5

Prep time: 35 min

Ingredients:

6 medium potatoes, chopped

1 leek, white part only, chopped

1 carrot, chopped

1 zucchini, peeled and chopped

1 celery stalk, chopped

3 cups water

1 cup soy milk

2 tbsp flaxseed

3 tbsp extra virgin olive oil

salt and black pepper, to taste

Directions:

Gently heat olive oil in a deep saucepan and sauté the onion for 2-3 minutes. Add in potatoes, carrot, zucchini and celery and cook for 2-3 minutes, stirring. Add in water and salt, and bring to a boil then lower heat and simmer until the vegetables are tender.

Blend until smooth; add soy milk, flaxseed, blend some more and serve.

Lentil, Barley and Kale Soup

Serves: 4-5

Prep time: 45 min

Ingredients:

2 medium leeks, chopped

3 garlic cloves, chopped

2 bay leaves

1 can tomatoes (15 oz), diced and undrained

1/2 cup red lentils

1/2 cup barley

1 bunch kale (10 oz), stemmed and coarsely chopped

4 cups water

3 tbsp extra virgin olive oil

1 tsp paprika

½ tsp cumin

Directions:

Heat oil in a large saucepan over medium-high heat. Sauté leeks and garlic until just fragrant. Add cumin and paprika, tomatoes, lentils, barley, and water. Season with salt and pepper.

Cover and bring to the boil then reduce heat and simmer for 40 minutes or until barley is tender. Add in kale, stir it in, and let it simmer for five minutes more.

Mediterranean Lentil Soup

Serves: 4-5

Prep time: 40 min

Ingredients:

1/2 cup red lentils

2 carrots, chopped

1 onion, chopped

1 garlic clove, chopped

1 small red pepper, chopped

1 can tomatoes, chopped

½ can chickpeas, drained

½ can white beans, drained

1 celery stalk, chopped

6 cups water

1 tbsp paprika

1 tsp ginger, grated

1 tsp cumin

3 tbsp extra virgin olive oil

Directions:

Heat olive oil in a deep soup pot and gently sauté onions, garlic, red pepper and ginger. Add in water, lentils, chickpeas, white beans, tomatoes, carrots, celery, and cumin.

Bring to a boil then lower heat and simmer for 35 minutes, or until the lentils are tender. Purée half the soup in a food processor.

Return the puréed soup to the pot, stir and serve.

Pea, Dill and Brown Rice Soup

Serves: 4

Prep time: 20 min

Ingredients:

1 (16 oz) bag frozen green peas

1 onion, chopped

3-4 garlic cloves, chopped

1/4 cup brown rice

3 tbsp fresh dill, chopped

3 tbsp extra virgin olive oil

1/2 cup fresh dill, finely chopped, to serve

salt and pepper, to taste

Directions:

Heat oil in a large saucepan over medium-high heat and sauté onion and garlic for 3-4 minutes.

Add in peas and vegetable broth and bring to the boil. Stir in rice, cover, reduce heat, and simmer for 35 minutes.

Season with salt and pepper and serve sprinkled with fresh dill.

Minted Pea and Nettle Soup

Serves: 4

Prep time: 20 min

Ingredients:

1 onion, chopped

3-4 garlic cloves, chopped

4 cups vegetable broth

2 tbsp dried mint leaves

1 16 oz bag frozen green peas

about 20 nettle tops

3 tbsp extra virgin olive oil

1 cup fresh dill, finely chopped, to serve

Directions:

Heat oil in a large saucepan over medium-high heat and sauté onion and garlic for 3-4 minutes.

Add in dried mint, peas, washed nettles, and vegetable broth and bring to the boil. Cover, reduce heat, and simmer for 15 minutes.

Remove from heat and set aside to cool slightly, then blend in batches, until smooth. Return soup to saucepan over medium-low heat and cook until heated through. Season with salt and pepper. Serve sprinkled with fresh dill.

Bean and Spinach Soup

Serves: 4-5

Prep time: 20 min

Ingredients:

1 onion, chopped

1 large carrot, chopped

2 garlic cloves, minced

1 15 oz can white beans, rinsed and drained

1 cup spinach leaves, trimmed and washed

3 cups vegetable broth

1 tbsp paprika

1 tbsp dried mint

3 tbsp extra virgin olive oil

salt and black pepper, to taste

Directions:

Heat the olive oil over medium heat and gently sauté the onion, garlic and carrot. Add in beans, broth, salt and pepper and bring to a boil.

Reduce heat and cook for 15 minutes, or until the carrots are tender. Stir in spinach, and simmer for about 5 minutes, until spinach wilts.

Mushroom and Kale Soup

Serves: 4-5

Prep time: 30 min

Ingredients:

1 onion, chopped

1 carrot, chopped

1 zucchini, peeled and diced

1 potato, peeled and diced

10 white mushrooms, chopped

1 bunch kale (10 oz), stemmed and coarsely chopped

3 cups vegetable broth

4 tbsp extra virgin olive oil

salt and black pepper. to taste

Directions:

Gently heat olive oil in a large soup pot. Add in onions, carrot and mushrooms and cook for 10-15 min or until vegetables are tender.

Add in vegetable broth, zucchini and kale. Season to taste with salt and pepper, and simmer for 20 minutes more.

Quinoa, Sweet Potato and Tomato Soup

Serves: 4

Prep time: 25 min

Ingredients:

½ cup quinoa

1 onion, chopped

1 large sweet potato, peeled and chopped

½ cup canned chickpeas, drained

1 cup baby spinach leaves

1 can tomatoes, drained and diced

3 cups vegetable broth

1 cup water

2 cloves garlic, chopped

1 tbsp grated fresh ginger

1 tsp cumin

1 tbsp paprika

2 tbsp extra virgin olive oil

Directions:

Wash quinoa very well, drain and set aside.

In a large soup pot, heat the olive oil over medium heat. Add the onions and garlic and sauté about 1-2 minutes, stirring. Add the sweet potato and sauté for another minute then add in the paprika, ginger and cumin.

Add water and broth, bring to a boil and stir in quinoa and

tomatoes.

Reduce heat to low, cover, and simmer for about 15 minutes, or until the sweet potatoes are tender. Season with salt and black pepper to taste. Blend the soup and return to the pot. Add the chickpeas and heat through, then add the spinach and cook until it wilts.

Red Lentil and Quinoa Soup

Serves: 4

Prep time: 35 min

Ingredients:

½ cup quinoa

1 cup red lentils

5 cups water

1 onion, chopped

2-3 garlic cloves, chopped

½ red bell pepper, finely cut

1 small tomato, chopped

3 tbsp extra virgin olive oil

1 tsp ginger

1 tsp cummin

1 tbsp paprika

salt and black pepper, to taste

Directions:

Wash and drain quinoa and red lentils and set aside.

In a large soup pot, heat the olive oil over medium heat. Add in the onion, garlic and red pepper and sauté for 1-2 minutes, stirring. Add the paprika and spices and stir. Add in the red lentils and quinoa, stir and add the water. Gently bring to the boil, then lower heat and simmer, covered for 25 minutes.

Add the tomato and cook for five more minutes. Blend the soup, serve and enjoy!

Spinach and Quinoa Soup

Serves: 4-5

Prep time: 20 min

Ingredients:

½ cup quinoa

1 onion, chopped

1 garlic clove, chopped

1 small zucchini, peeled and diced

1 tomato, diced

2 cups fresh spinach, cut

4 cups water

3 tbsp extra virgin olive oil

1 tbsp paprika

salt and pepper, to taste

Directions:

Heat olive oil in a deep soup pot over medium-high heat. Add onion and garlic and sauté for 1 minute, stirring constantly. Add in paprika and zucchini, stir, and cook for 2-3 minutes more.

Add 4 cups of water and bring to a boil then add in spinach and quinoa. Stir and reduce heat. Simmer for 15 minutes then set aside to cool.

Vegetable Quinoa Soup

Serves: 4-5

Prep time: 25 min

Ingredients:

½ cup quinoa

1 cup sliced leeks

1 garlic clove, chopped

½ carrot, diced

1 tomato, diced

1 small zucchini, diced

½ cup frozen green beans

4 cups water

1 tsp paprika

4 tbsp extra virgin olive oil

5-6 tbsp lemon juice, to serve

Directions:

Wash quinoa in a fine sieve under running water until the water runs clear. Set aside to drain.

Heat olive oil in a soup pot and gently sauté the leeks, garlic and carrot for 1 minute, stirring. Add in paprika, zucchini, tomatoes, green beans and water.

Bring to a boil, add quinoa and lower heat to medium-low. Simmer for 20 minutes, or until the vegetables are tender. Serve with lemon juice.

Kale, Leek and Quinoa Soup

Serves: 4-5

Prep time: 35 min

Ingredients:

½ cup quinoa

2 leeks, white part only, chopped

1/2 onion, chopped

1 can tomatoes, diced and undrained

1 bunch kale (10 oz), stemmed and coarsely chopped

4 cups vegetable broth

3 tbsp extra virgin olive oil

salt and pepper, to taste

Directions:

Heat olive oil in a large pot over medium heat and gently sauté the onion for 3-4 minutes. Add in the leeks, season with salt and pepper, and add the vegetable broth, tomatoes and quinoa.

Bring to a boil then reduce heat and simmer for 15 minutes. Stir in kale and cook for another 5 minutes.

Main Dish Recipes

Chicken and Zucchini Frittata

Serves: 4

Prep time: 30 min

Ingredients:

1 cup chicken, chopped finely

1/2 onion, finely chopped

2 garlic cloves, chopped

1 zucchini, peeled and diced

1 tomato, diced

2 tbsp dill, finely chopped

4 eggs

3 tbsp soy milk

4 tbsp olive oil

Directions:

Heat two tablespoons of olive oil in a frying pan and gently cook the chicken until almost cooked through. Add the onion and garlic and cook for another minute. Set aside.

In the same pan, heat the remaining olive oil. Cook the zucchini and tomato for for 3-4 minutes, until lightly cooked. Add in the chicken and mix everything well. Pour it all into the baking dish.

In a medium bowl, whisk eggs, soy milk and dill together. Pour over the top of the chicken and vegetable mixture, making sure that it covers it well. Bake in a preheated to 360 F oven for around 15 minutes, until set. Garnish with fresh dill.

Hearty Chicken Spinach Frittata

Serves: 4

Prep time: 30 min

Ingredients:

1 cup chicken, chopped finely

3-4 green onions, finely chopped

5 oz frozen chopped spinach, defrosted and excess moisture squeezed out

½ zucchini, peeled and shredded

1 large tomato, thinly sliced

2 tbsp fresh rosemary leaves, finely chopped

4 eggs

3 tbsp flaxseed

6 tbsp milk

4 tbsp olive oil

Directions:

Grease a shallow casserole dish. Heat two tablespoons of olive oil in a frying pan and gently cook the chicken until almost cooked through. Add in the onions and garlic and cook for another minute. Set aside.

In the same pan, heat the remaining olive oil. Cook the zucchini and spinach, stirring constantly, until lightly cooked. Add in the chicken mixture, and combine everything well. Pour it all into the casserole.

In a medium bowl, whisk eggs, flaxseed, milk and rosemary together. Pour over the top of the chicken and vegetable mixture, making sure that it covers it well. Lay the tomato slices on top.

Bake in a preheated to 360 F oven for around 15 minutes, until set. Garnish with rosemary.

Chicken and Mushroom Frittata

Serves: 4

Prep time: 20 min

Ingredients:

1 cup cooked chicken meat, chopped

1 cup white mushrooms, chopped

½ onion, chopped or 2 spring onions, chopped

1 garlic clove, chopped

1 large tomato, thinly sliced

1/2 tsp salt

1/2 tsp black pepper

1 tsp dried thyme

4 large eggs, beaten well

2 tbsp extra virgin olive oil

Directions:

Grease a shallow casserole dish. Heat two tablespoons of olive oil in a frying pan and gently cook the onions and garlic until onion is transparent. Add in the mushrooms, stir, and cook on medium-high heat for 3-4 minutes. Add in the chicken and combine everything well. Pour it into the casserole.

In a medium bowl, whisk eggs, salt, black pepper and thyme together. Pour over the top of the chicken and mushroom mixture, making sure that it covers it well.

Lay the tomato slices on top. Bake in a preheated to 360 F oven for around 15 minutes, until set.

Greek Style Chicken Skewers

Serves: 4

Prep time: 50 min

Ingredients:

2 lbs chicken breasts, diced

3 small zucchinis, diced

12 white button mushrooms

3 tbsp extra virgin olive oil

1 lemon, juiced

2 garlic cloves, crushed

1 tsp dried oregano

1 tsp dried rosemary

12 wooden skewers

Directions:

Thread chicken, mushrooms and zucchinis alternately onto each of 12 skewers. Place in a shallow dish. Combine extra virgin olive oil and lemon juice, garlic and oregano. Pour over chicken. Turn to coat. Marinate for at least 30 minutes.

Preheat a barbecue plate on medium-high heat. Cook skewers for 4 minutes each side or until chicken is just cooked through.

Chicken Puttanesca

Serves: 4

Prep time: 30 min

Ingredients:

4 boneless chicken breasts

2 tbsp extra virgin olive oil

for the sauce:

2 tbsp extra virgin olive oil

4 garlic cloves, crushed

1 small onion, diced

1/2 cup green olives, pitted and chopped

2 tbsp capers, drained and coarsely chopped

3 boneless anchovy filets, coarsely chopped

2 tomatoes, diced

1 tbsp tomato paste

2 tbsp flaxseed

1/2 tsp paprika

salt and black pepper, to taste

Directions:

Heat two tablespoons of olive oil in a large skillet and brown the chicken for about 2 minutes, each side. Cover with a lid and cook for about 10-15 minutes, or until cooked through. Set aside on 4 plates.

In the same skillet, heat two tablespoons of olive oil. Add in garlic, onions, anchovies, olives, capers and paprika. Gently sauté these ingredients, stirring constantly, for about one minute.

Add in the tomatoes and tomato paste, season with salt and pepper, add the flaxseed and cook over high heat for 5-6 minutes or until the tomatoes are cooked and the sauce thickens. Divide the sauce between the chicken breasts and serve.

Spinach with Ground Beef and Tofu

Serves: 4

Prep time: 30 min

Ingredients:

1 cup ground beef

1 cup tofu, crumbled

5 cups fresh spinach, chopped

1/2 cup canned tomatoes, drained, cubed

1/2 onion, finely chopped

1/4 cup brown rice

4 tbsp extra virgin olive oil

1 tbsp paprika

salt, to taste

black pepper, to taste

Directions:

In a large sauce pan heat olive oil and gently sauté the onion for about 2-3 minutes. Add in the ground beef, crumbled tofu, paprika, salt and black pepper and cook, stirring, until the ground beef turns brown.

Add in rice and tomatoes and simmer, covered, for 30 minutes.

Stir in spinach and cook until it wilts.

Ground Beef and Lentil Casserole

Serves: 4-5

Prep time: 30 min

Ingredients:

1 lb ground beef

1 small onion, chopped

2 garlic cloves, crushed

1 cup dry green lentils

1 carrot, chopped

2 cups water

2 bay leaves

1 tsp dried oregano

1 tbsp paprika

1/2 tsp salt

1/2 tsp cumin

3 tbsp extra virgin olive oil

black pepper, to taste

Directions:

Heat the olive oil in a casserole over medium-high heat. Add the onion and carrot and sauté for 4-5 minutes. Add in garlic and sauté a minute more.

Add the ground beef and cook for 4-5 minutes, stirring, until browned. Add the paprika, cumin, oregano, bay leaves, tomatoes, lentils and water.

Bring everything to a boil then reduce heat and simmer for 20 minutes, or until the beef is cooked through. Remove the bay leaves and serve.

Salmon Kebabs

Serves: 4-5

Prep time: 30 min

Ingredients:

2 shallots, ends trimmed, halved

2 zucchinis, cut in 2 inch cubes

1 cup cherry tomatoes

6 skinless salmon fillets, cut into 1 inch pieces

3 limes, cut into thin wedges

Directions:

Preheat barbecue or char grill on medium-high. Thread fish cubes onto skewers, then zucchinis, shallots and tomatoes. Repeat to make 12 kebabs. Bake the kebabs for about 3 minutes each side for medium cooked.

Transfer to a plate, cover with foil and set aside for 5 minutes to rest.

Mediterranean Baked Salmon

Serves: 4-5

Prep time: 35 min

Ingredients:

2 (6 oz) boneless salmon fillets

1 tomato, thinly sliced

1 onion, thinly sliced

1 tbsp capers

3 tbsp olive oil

1 tsp dry oregano

3 tbsp Parmesan cheese

salt and black pepper, to taste

Directions:

Preheat oven to 350 F. Place the salmon fillets in a baking dish, sprinkle with oregano, top with onion and tomato slices, drizzle with olive oil, and sprinkle with capers and Parmesan cheese.

Cover the dish with foil and bake for 30 minutes, or until the fish flakes easily.

Simple Oven-Baked Sea Bass

Serves: 4

Prep time: 35 min

Ingredients:

1 lb sea bass (cleaned and scaled

5 oz fennel, trimmed and sliced

5-6 spring onions, chopped

2 garlic cloves, chopped

10 black olives, pitted and halved

2-3 lemon wedges

1 tbsp capers

2 garlic cloves, finely chopped

½ tsp paprika

½ cup dry white wine

3 tbsp extra virgin olive oil

salt and pepper, to taste

Directions:

In a cup, mix garlic, olive oil, salt, and black pepper.

Arrange the sliced fennel in a shallow oven-proof casserole. Add the green onions and lay the fish on top. Pour over the olive mixture. Scatter the olives, paprika and lemon wedges over the fish, then pour the wine over the top.

Cover the dish with a lid or foil and bake for 30 minutes, or until the fish flakes easily.

Potato, Pea and Cauliflower Curry

Serves: 4

Prep time: 25 min

Ingredients:

1 lb potatoes, peeled and cubed

1 lb cauliflower, cut into small florets

1 cup fresh peas

1 onion, finely chopped

2 garlic cloves, crushed

1 cup vegetable broth

1 tsp finely grated fresh ginger

1 tbsp curry powder

2 tbsp extra virgin olive oil

1/2 cup tomato pasta sauce

1/2 cup soy milk

1 tsp corn flour

Directions:

Heat oil in a large saucepan over medium heat. Add the onion and gently saute, stirring, for 3-4 minutes until transparent. Add in garlic and ginger, and cook for 1 minute until just fragrant.

Add in the curry powder, potatoes and cauliflower florets, and stir. Add in broth and tomato sauce and simmer, uncovered, for 15-20 minutes or until the potatoes are tender.

Combine the soy milk and cornflour in a small bowl. Gradually add to the potato mixture, stirring constantly. Add the peas, reduce heat, and simmer for 2 minutes or until the peas are tender and the mixture is heated through. Serve with rice.

Cauliflower with Chilli and Mustard

Serves: 4

Prep time: 25 min

Ingredients:

2 lbs cauliflower, cut into small florets

3 long fresh green chillies, thinly sliced

1 onion, finely chopped

2 garlic cloves, crushed

1/2 cup vegetable broth

2 teaspoons mustard seeds

1 tsp ground tumeric

1 tsp tamarind paste

2 tbsp extra virgin olive oil

Directions:

Heat oil in a large saucepan over medium heat. Add the onion and gently saute, stirring, for 3-4 minutes until transparent. Add in garlic and chilli, and cook for 1 minute until just fragrant. Add the mustard seeds and turmeric and saute, stirring, for 20 seconds or until the mustard seeds pop.

Add the cauliflower and stir to coat. Add the vegetable broth and tamarind paste and simmer for 4 minutes or until the cauliflower is tender crisp. Season with salt to taste ans serve.

Baked Cauliflower

Serves: 4

Prep time: 25 min

Ingredients:

1 small cauliflower, cut into florets

1 tbsp garlic powder

1 tsp paprika

salt, to taste

black pepper, to taste

4 tbsp extra virgin olive oil

Directions:

Combine olive oil, paprika, salt, pepper and garlic powder together. Toss in the cauliflower florets and place in a baking dish in one layer. Bake in a preheated to 350 F oven for 20 minutes or until golden.

Maple Roast Parsnip with Pear and Sage

Serves: 4

Prep time: 65 min

Ingredients:

5 parsnips, peeled, halved, cut into large wedges

2 large pears, cut into wedges

1 large onion, cut into wedges

1 tbsp garlic powder

1/3 cup fresh sage leaves

2 tablespoons maple syrup

1/4 teaspoon dried chilli flakes

4 tbsp extra virgin olive oil

Directions:

Preheat oven to 350F. Line 2 baking trays with baking paper. Place the parsnip, pear, onion, and sage on the prepared trays.

Combine the maple syrup, olive oil, garlic powder and dried chilli flakes in a bowl.

Pour the maple mixture evenly over the parsnip mixture and gently toss to combine. Bake, turning halfway during cooking, for 1 hour or until the parsnip is golden and tender.

Balsamic Roasted Carrots and Baby Onions

Serves: 4

Prep time: 50 min

Ingredients:

2 bunches baby carrots, scrubbed, ends trimmed

10 small onions, peeled, halved

4 tbsp brown sugar

1 tsp thyme

2 tbsp extra virgin olive oil

Directions:

Preheat oven to 350F. Line a baking tray with baking paper.

Place the carrots, onion, thyme and oil in a large bowl and toss until well coated. Arrange carrots and onion, in a single layer, on the baking tray. Roast for 25 minutes or until tender.

Sprinkle over the sugar and vinegar and toss to coat. Roast for 25-30 minutes more or until vegetables are tender and caramelized. Season with salt and pepper to taste and serve.

Potato and Zucchini Bake

Serves: 5-6

Prep time: 25 min

Ingredients:

1 lb potatoes, peeled and sliced

4-5 zucchinis, peeled and sliced

1 onion, sliced

2 garlic cloves, crushed

½ cup water

4 tbsp extra virgin olive oil

1 tsp dry oregano

1/3 cup fresh dill, chopped

salt and black pepper, to taste

Directions:

Place the potatoes, zucchinis and onion in a shallow ovenproof baking dish. Pour over the olive oil and water. Add salt, black pepper to taste, and toss everything together.

Bake in a preheated to 350 F oven for 40 minutes, stirring halfway through, bake for 5 minutes more and serve.

Creamy Avocado and Chicken Spaghetti

Serves: 5-6

Prep time: 20 min

Ingredients:

12 oz whole-wheat spaghetti

1 cup cooked chicken, shredded

2 avocados, peeled and diced

1 cup cherry tomatoes, halved

1 garlic clove, chopped

2 tbsp basil pesto

5 tbsp olive oil

4 tbsp lemon juice

1/4 cup grated Parmesan cheese

Directions:

In a large pot of boiling salted water, cook spaghetti according to package instructions. Drain and set aside in a large bowl.

In a blender, combine lemon juice, garlic, basil pesto and avocados and blend until smooth.

Combine spaghetti, chicken, cherry tomatoes and avocado sauce. Sprinkle with Parmesan cheese and serve immediately.

Easy Summer Spaghetti

Serves: 5-6

Prep time: 20 min

Ingredients:

12 oz whole-wheat spaghetti

2-3 spring onions, finely cut

1 small zucchini, peeled and diced

1 small eggplant, peeled and diced

1/2 cup canned chickpeas, drained

1/2 cup black olives, pitted and halved

2 garlic cloves, crushed

1.5 cups tomato sauce

2 cups water

3 tbsp extra virgin olive oil

1 tsp dried basil

1/3 cup fresh parsley, finely cut

1 tsp salt

Directions:

Heat a deep saucepan over medium-high heat. Add in olive oil and gently saute the spring onion and garlic for 1 minute, stirring. Add in the olives, chickpeas, eggplant, zucchini, water, tomato sauce, basil, and season with salt and black pepper.

Bring to a boil, add spaghetti and stir. Reduce heat and cook until the spaghetti is cooked to al dente. Sprinkle with parsley, adjust seasonings, and serve.

One-pot Lentil and Olive Pasta

Serves: 5-6

Prep time: 20 min

Ingredients:

12 oz small whole-wheat pasta

1/2 small onion, chopped

1/2 celery stalk, finely chopped

1 can lentils, rinsed, drained

1/2 cup green olives, pitted and halved

2-3 garlic cloves, crushed

2 cups tomato sauce

2 cups water

1/2 tsp cumin

3 tbsp extra virgin olive oil

1/2 cup fresh mint, finely cut

1 cup feta cheese, crumbled

Directions:

Heat a deep saucepan over medium-high heat. Add in olive oil and gently saute the onion and celery. Add in garlic, lentils, olives, water, tomato sauce, and cumin and season with salt and black pepper to taste.

Bring to a boil, then add pasta and stir. Reduce heat and simmer until the spaghetti is cooked to al dente. Sprinkle with feta and mint, and serve.

Summer Zucchini and Tofu Risotto

Serves: 4-5

Prep time: 20 min

Ingredients:

2 medium zucchinis, peeled and diced

5-6 spring onions, finely cut

1 medium tomato, diced

1 cup risotto rice

1/2 cup frozen peas

1/2 cup sweet corn

2 1/2 cups vegetable broth

10 oz tofu, crumbled

2 tbsp extra virgin olive oil

1 tsp salt

1 bunch fresh dill

Directions:

In a deep saucepan, heat olive oil and gently sauté the green onions for 1-2 minutes. Add in zucchinis, tomato, peas, sweet corn, rice, salt, and half the vegetable broth.

Stir and cook for 10 mins or until the liquid has evaporated, stirring from time to time. Add in the rest of the vegetable broth and the crumbled tofu and cook for 5-6 min more. Sprinkle with dill and serve.

Vegetable Quinoa Stew

Serves: 4-5

Prep time: 20 min

Ingredients:

1 cup quinoa

1 ½ cup water

1 onion, finely cut

2 red bell peppers, chopped

1 zucchini, peeled and chopped

1 cup fresh green peas

1 tomato, chopped

2 garlic cloves, chopped

1 tbsp paprika

3 tbsp extra virgin olive oil

salt, to taste

½ cup fresh dill, finely cut, to serve

Directions:

Rinse the quinoa very well in a sieve under running water and set aside to drain.

Heat olive oil in large saucepan over medium-high heat. Add the onion and sauté for 1-2 minutes. Add in the garlic, paprika, bell pepper, green peas and zucchini. Cook, stirring occasionally, for 5 minutes then add the tomato and the water.

Bring to the boil and add quinoa. Stir, cover, and cook for 15 minutes. Season with salt to taste and serve sprinkled with dill.

Eggplant and Qinoa Stew

Serves: 4-5

Prep time: 20 min

Ingredients:

1 cup quinoa

1 ½ cups water

1 large eggplant, peeled and diced

1 cup canned tomatoes, drained and diced

1 zucchini, diced

5-6 black olives, pitted and halved

1 onion, chopped

4 garlic cloves, chopped

1 tbsp tomato paste

3 tbsp extra virgin olive oil

1 tsp paprika

½ cup parsley leaves, finely cut, to serve

Directions:

Rinse the quinoa very well in a fine sieve under running water and set aside to drain.

Gently sauté onions, garlic and eggplant in olive oil on medium-high heat for 5-6 minutes. Add in paprika and tomato paste and stir for 1-2 minutes.

Add in the rest of the vegetables and the water; and bring to the boil. Stir in quinoa, lower heat and simmer, covered, for 15 minutes. Sprinkle with parsley and serve.

Comforting Quinoa Shepherd's Stew

Serves: 4-5

Prep time: 20 min

Ingredients:

1 cup quinoa

1 ½ cups water

1 onion, finely cut

2 garlic cloves, chopped

2 red peppers, chopped

2 carrots, chopped

1 large potato, diced

6-7 white mushrooms, chopped

1-2 tomatoes, diced

2 tbsp extra virgin olive oil

1 tbsp paprika

1 bay leaf

1 tbsp thyme

1 tsp summer savory

Directions:

Wash quinoa very well, drain and set aside.

In a large soup pot or casserole dish, heat the oil over medium heat. Add the onion, bell peppers and garlic and sauté until softened, about 3 minutes. Stir in the paprika. bay leaf, thyme and savory and stir.

Add the other vegetables and mushrooms and cook for 1-2

minutes, stirring. Add in water and bring to the boil then stir in the quinoa. Reduce heat to low and simmer, covered, for 15-20 minutes.

Easy Moroccan Vegetable Stew with Quinoa

Serves: 6

Prep time: 20 min

Ingredients:

1 large onion, chopped

2 garlic cloves, chopped

1 cup quinoa

2 cups vegetable broth

1 cup canned chickpeas, drained

1 cup canned tomatoes, diced and undrained

1 carrot, chopped

1 cup baby spinach leaves

¼ cup dried prunes

¼ cup dried apricots

1 zucchini, quartered lengthwise and chopped

½ cup almonds, coarsely chopped

3 tbsp extra virgin olive oil

1 tsp grated ginger

1 tsp ground cinnamon

Directions:

In a large soup pot or casserole dish, heat the oil over medium heat. Add the onion, ginger, garlic and cinnamon and sauté for 2-3 minutes, or until the onion has softened.

Add in the vegetable broth, chickpeas, tomatoes, carrots, apricots and prunes and bring to a boil. Stir in add quinoa and zucchinis, reduce heat and simmer, covered, for 15 minutes.

Add in the baby spinach and cook until it wilts. Add the almonds, stir and serve.

Zucchini and Buckwheat Stew

Serves: 4-5

Prep time: 20 min

Ingredients:

1 cup toasted buckwheat groats

1 ½ cups vegetable broth

1 onion, finely chopped

3 garlic cloves, chopped

4 zucchinis, peeled and diced

1 cup fresh dill, finely cut

3 tbsp extra virgin olive oil

salt, to taste

Directions:

In a deep saucepan, heat olive oil and gently sauté the onion and garlic for 1-2 minutes. Add the diced zucchinis and sauté for 5-6 minutes, stirring.

Add in vegetable broth and bring to the boil. Stir in the toasted buckwheat, finely cut dill and salt to taste, and simmer for 15-20 minutes.

Power Buckwheat Stew

Serves: 4-5

Prep time: 20 min

Ingredients:

1 cup toasted buckwheat groats

1 cup vegetable broth or water

1 onion, chopped

1 potato, chopped

1 zucchini, peeled and chopped

1 tomato, diced

½ cup frozen corn kernels

½ cup frozen peas

½ cup black olives, halved, pitted

2 garlic cloves, minced

4 tbsp extra virgin olive oil

salt and pepper, to taste

1 cup parsley, finely cut

Directions:

In a deep saucepan, heat olive oil and gently sauté the onion and garlic for a minute. Add in the green peas, potato, zucchini, corn, olives and cook, stirring for 3-4 minutes.

Add water or vegetable broth and bring to the boil. Stir in the diced tomato and the toasted buckwheat. Reduce heat, cover, and simmer for 10 minutes, stirring occasionally. Serve sprinkled with parsley and enjoy!

Quick Buckwheat Chilli

Serves: 4-5

Prep time: 20-25 min

Ingredients:

1 cup toasted buckwheat groats

1 ¾ cups vegetable broth

1 large onion, finely cut

3 cloves garlic, chopped

1 green bell pepper, chopped

1 can diced tomatoes

1 can mixed beans, well rinsed and drained

1 tbsp paprika

1 tsp chilli powder

1 tsp ground cumin

2 tbsp extra virgin olive oil

¼ cup chopped fresh coriander, to serve

Directions:

In a large soup pot or casserole dish, heat the oil over medium heat. Add the onion, bell pepper and garlic and sauté until softened, about 3 minutes. Stir in the chilli powder, cumin and paprika and sauté for another minute. Add the buckwheat and stir to combine well.

Stir in the tomatoes, beans and vegetable broth. Bring to a boil then reduce heat to low and simmer, covered, for about 20 minutes. Serve sprinkled with fresh coriander.

Spicy Chickpea, Tofu and Spinach Stew

Serves: 4

Prep time: 40 min

Ingredients:

1 onion, chopped

3 garlic cloves, chopped

1 15 oz can chickpeas, drained and rinsed

10 oz extra-firm tofu, cubed

1 15 oz can tomatoes, diced and undrained

1 1 lb bag baby spinach

a handful of blanched almonds

½ cup vegetable broth

1 tbsp hot chilli paste

½ tsp cumin

salt and pepper, to taste

Directions:

Heat olive oil in a large saucepan over medium-high heat. Gently sauté onion and garlic for 4-5 minutes, or until tender. Add spices and stir. Add in tofu, chickpeas, tomatoes, almonds and broth.

Bring to a boil, then reduce heat to low and simmer, partially covered, for 10 minutes. Add the chilli paste and spinach to the pot and stir until the spinach wilts. Remove from heat and season with salt and pepper to taste.

Moroccan Chickpea Stew

Serves: 4-5

Prep time: 20 min

Ingredients:

1 onion, chopped

3 garlic cloves, chopped

2 large carrots, chopped

2 sweet potatoes, peeled and chopped

4-5 dates, pitted and chopped

1 cup spinach, chopped

1 15 oz can tomatoes, diced and undrained

1 15 oz can chickpeas, rinsed and drained

1 cup vegetable broth

1 tbsp ground cumin

½ tsp chilli powder

½ tsp ground turmeric

½ teaspoon salt

3 tbsp extra virgin olive oil

½ cup chopped cilantro, to serve

grated lemon zest, to serve

Directions:

Heat olive oil in a large saucepan over medium-high heat. Gently sauté onion, garlic and carrots for 4-5 minutes, or until tender. Add all spices and stir. Stir in all other ingredients except the spinach.

Bring to a boil, cover, reduce heat, and simmer for 20 minutes, or until potatoes are tender. Add in spinach, stir and cook it until it wilts. Serve over brown rice, quinoa or couscous and top with chopped cilantro and lemon zest.

Chickpea, Rice and Mushroom Stew

Serves: 4-5

Prep time: 20-30 min

Ingredients:

1 15 oz can chickpeas, drained

1 large onion, finely cut

2 cups mushrooms, chopped

2 carrots, chopped

1 15 oz can tomatoes, diced, undrained

1/3 cup rice, washed

1 cup vegetable broth

4 tbsp extra virgin olive oil

1 tsp oregano

1 tbsp paprika

1 cup fresh parsley, finely cut

1 tbsp sugar

Directions:

In a deep, heavy-bottomed saucepan, heat olive oil and gently sauté the onion and carrots for 4-5 minutes, stirring constantly. Add in paprika, chickpeas, rice, mushrooms, tomatoes, sugar and vegetable broth and stir again.

Season with salt, oregano, ground black pepper and bring to the boil. Cover, reduce heat, and simmer for about 20 minutes, stirring from time to time. Sprinkle with parsley, simmer for a minute more and serve.

Easy Chickpea Dinner

Serves: 4-5

Prep time: 20 min

Ingredients:

1 large onion, chopped

15-20 black olives, pitted

2 zucchinis, peeled and diced

1 15 oz can chickpeas, drained

1 cup marinara sauce

1/2 cup fresh parsley leaves, finely cut

4 tbsp extra virgin olive oil

salt and black pepper, to taste

Directions:

In a deep saucepan, heat olive oil and sauté the onion for 2-3 minutes.

Add in the chickpeas, zucchinis, olives and marinara sauce. Season with black pepper, and simmer on medium-high for 30 minutes. Sprinkle with parsley and serve.

Baked Beans and Rice Casserole

Serves: 4-5

Prep time: 30 min

Ingredients:

2 cans (15 oz) white or red beans, drained

1 cup water or vegetable broth

2/3 cup rice

2 onions, chopped

1 cup parsley, finely cut

7-8 fresh mint leaves, finely cut

3 tbsp extra virgin olive oil

1 tbsp paprika

½ tsp black pepper

1 tsp salt

Directions:

Heat olive oil in an ovenproof casserole dish and gently sauté the chopped onions for 1-2 minutes. Stir in paprika and rice and cook, stirring constantly, for another minute.

Add in beans and a cup of water or vegetable broth, season with salt and black pepper, stir in mint and parsley, and bake in a preheated to 350 F oven for 20 minutes.

Green Peas and Rice Casserole

Serves: 4-5

Prep time: 20 min

Ingredients:

1 onion, chopped

1 1 lb bag frozen peas

3 garlic cloves, chopped

3-4 mushrooms, chopped

2/3 cup white rice

1 cup water

4 tbsp extra virgin olive oil

salt and black pepper, to taste

Directions:

In a deep ovenproof casserole dish, heat olive oil and sauté the onions, garlic and mushrooms for 2-3 minutes. Add in the rice and cook, stirring constantly for 1 minute.

Add in a cup of warm water and the frozen peas, stir, bake in a preheated to 350 F oven for 20 minutes, and serve.

Green Beans and Potatoes

Serves: 4-4

Prep time: 20 min

Ingredients:

1 bag frozen green beans

3 potatoes, peeled and diced

1 tsp tomato paste

1 carrot, sliced

1 onion, chopped

2 garlic cloves, crushed

3 tbsp extra virgin olive oil

1/2 cup fresh dill, finely chopped

½ cup water

1 tsp paprika

salt and pepper, to taste

Directions:

Heat olive oil in a deep saucepan and sauté the onion for 2-3 minutes, stirring. Add in garlic and saute until just fragrant. Add in the green beans, and all remaining ingredients.

Stir to combine very well, cover, and simmer for about 20-30 minutes until all vegetables are tender. Serve warm sprinkled with fresh dill.

Delicious Mushroom Tofu Pizza

Serves: 4

Prep time: 25 min

Ingredients:

1 store-bought or homemade dough

2-3 spring onions, chopped

10 white mushrooms, chopped

1 red bell pepper, chopped

1/2 cup tomato sauce

1 cup tofu pieces

2 tbsp olive oil

1/2 tsp oregano

1 tsp thyme

1/2 tsp garlic powder

salt and black pepper, to taste

2-3 cups mozzarella cheese, shredded

Directions:

In a large skillet, heat olive oil and gently sauté spring onions and bell pepper for 4-5 minutes until slightly charred. Add in the tofu pieces, mushrooms, garlic powder, oregano and thyme and sauté for 5 minutes more. Season with salt and black pepper to taste.

Roll out dough onto a floured surface and transfer to a round baking sheet lined with parchment paper or an oiled pizza stone.

Top with tomato sauce and the sautéed tofu and mushroom mixture. Sprinkle with shredded mozzarella cheese.

Bake for about 15 minutes, until the crust is golden brown and the cheese is completely melted. Let rest for 3-4 minutes before cutting, then serve immediately.

Breakfast and Dessert Recipes

Avocado and Feta Toast with Poached Eggs

Serves: 4

Prep time: 5 min

Ingredients:

1 avocado, peeled and chopped

½ cup feta cheese, crumbled

2 tbsp chopped fresh mint

1 tsp lime juice

½ tsp cumin

4 thick slices rye bread, lightly toasted

4 poached eggs

Directions:

Mash avocados with a fork until almost smooth. Add the feta, fresh mint, lime juice and cumin. Season with salt and pepper to taste. Stir to combine.

Toast 4 slices of rye bread until golden. Spoon 1/4 of the avocado mixture onto each slice of bread. Top with a poached egg and serve immediately.

Avocado and Olive Paste on Toasted Rye Bread

Serves: 4

Prep time: 5 min

Ingredients:

1 avocado, halved, peeled and finely chopped

1 tbsp green onions, finely chopped

2 tbsp green olive paste

1 tbsp lemon juice

Directions:

Mash avocados with a fork or potato masher until almost smooth. Add the onions, green olive paste and lemon juice. Season with salt and pepper to taste. Stir to combine.

Toast 4 slices of rye bread until golden. Spoon 1/4 of the avocado mixture onto each slice of bread.

Avocado, Lettuce and Tomato Sandwiches

Serves: 2

Prep time: 3-4 min

Ingredients:

4 slices rye bread

1 tbsp mayonnaise

1 tbsp basil pesto

2 large leaves lettuce

1/2 tomato, thinly sliced

1/2 avocado, peeled and sliced

6 very thin slices cucumber

Directions:

Combine mayonnaise and pesto. Spread this mixture on the four slices of bread.

Layer two slices with one lettuce leaf, two slices tomato, two slices avocado and three slices cucumber. Top with remaining bread slices. Cut sandwiches in half diagonally and serve.

Avocado and Chickpea Sandwiches

Serves: 4

Prep time: 3-4 min

Ingredients:

4 slices white bread

1/2 cup canned chickpeas

1 small avocado

2 green onions, finely chopped

1 egg, hard boiled

1/2 tomato, thinly sliced

1/2 cucumber, thinly sliced

salt, to taste

Directions:

Mash the avocado and chickpeas with a fork or potato masher until smooth. Add in green onions and salt and combine well.

Spread this mixture on the four slices of bread. Top each slice with tomato, cucumber and egg, and serve.

Quick Tofu and Vegetable Scramble

Serves: 4

Prep time: 10 min

Ingredients:

1/2 small onion, chopped

2 tomatoes, diced

1/4 cup fresh peas

6 eggs

12 oz tofu, crumbled

4 tbsp extra virgin olive oil

black pepper, to taste

salt, to taste

Directions:

In a large pan sauté onion over medium heat for 1-2 minutes, stirring. Add in tomatoes and peas and simmer until the peas are soft and the mixture is almost dry.

Add in tofu and eggs, stir, and cook until well mixed and not too liquid.

Season with black pepper and serve.

Raisin Quinoa Breakfast

Serves: 4

Prep time: 15 min

Ingredients:

1 cup quinoa

2 cups milk

2 tbsp walnuts, crushed

2 tbsp raisins

2 tbsp dried cranberries

2-3 tbsp honey, optional

½ tsp vanilla extract

1 tbsp chia seeds

Directions:

Rinse quinoa with cold water and drain. Place milk and quinoa into a saucepan and bring to a boil. Add vanilla. Reduce heat to low and simmer for about 15 minutes stirring from time to time.

Set aside to cool then serve in a bowl, topped with honey, chia seeds, raisins, cranberries and crushed walnuts.

Banana Cinnamon Fritters

Serves: 4

Prep time: 15 min

Ingredients:

1 cup self-raising flour

1 egg, beaten

3/4 cup sparkling water

2 tsp ground cinnamon

sunflower oil, for frying

2-3 bananas, cut diagonally into 4 pieces each

powdered sugar, to serve

Directions:

Sift flour and cinnamon into a bowl and make a well in the centre. Add egg and enough sparkling water to mix to a smooth batter.

Heat sunflower oil in a saucepan, enough to cover the base by 1-2 inch, so when a little batter dropped into the oil sizzles and rises to the surface. Dip banana pieces into the batter, then fry for 2-3 minutes or until golden.

Remove with a slotted spoon and drain on paper towels. Sprinkle with sugar and serve hot.

Avocado and Banana Muffins

Serves: 12

Prep time: 20 min

Ingredients:

1/2 cup mashed avocado

1/2 cup mashed bananas

2 large eggs

1/2 cup milk

2 cups all-purpose flour

1 cup sugar

1 tsp baking soda

1 tsp salt

1/2 cup chocolate chips

Directions:

Preheat oven to 375 F. Grease 12 muffin tin wells or line with paper cups.

In a large bowl, mix avocado, bananas, eggs and milk. In a separate bowl, whisk flour, sugar, baking soda and salt. Combine with avocado mixture; do not over-mix. Stir in chocolate chips.

Spoon batter into prepared muffin tin; bake 15-18 minutes or until tops start to brown and a toothpick inserted into a muffin comes out clean.

Avocado and Pumpkin Muffins

Serves: 13-14

Prep time: 20 min

Ingredients:

1/2 cup mashed avocado

1 1/2 cup pumpkin puree

2 large eggs

2 cups flour

1 cup sugar

1 tsp baking soda

1 tsp salt

1 tsp cinnamon

1 tsp vanilla

1/2 cup walnuts, chopped

Directions:

Preheat oven to 375 F. Grease 12 muffin tin wells or line with paper cups.

In a large bowl, mix avocado, pumpkin and eggs. In a separate bowl, whisk flour, sugar, baking soda, cinnamon, vanilla and salt. Combine with avocado mixture; do not over-mix. Stir in walnuts.

Spoon batter into prepared muffin tin; bake 15-18 minutes or until tops start to brown and a toothpick inserted into a muffin comes out clean.

Oatmeal Muffins

Serves: 13-14

Prep time: 20 min

Ingredients:

2 eggs, beaten

1 cup instant oatmeal

3/4 cup flour

1/2 cup sugar

1/2 tsp salt

2 tbsp flaxseed

1 tsp baking powder

1/2 tsp baking soda

1/2 tsp cinnamon

1/3 cup walnuts, crushed

1/4 cup raisins

1/2 cup vegetable oil

2/3 cup milk

1 tsp lemon zest

1 tsp vanilla extract

Directions:

Preheat the oven to 350 F and grease 12 muffin tin wells or line with paper cups.

Mix together the oats, sugar, flour, salt, baking soda, baking powder, flaxseed cinnamon, walnuts and raisins. In a separate bowl mix together the oil, milk, eggs, vanilla and lemon zest.

Pour the wet ingredients into the dry ingredients and stir for about 15 seconds, just to bring the ingredients together. Scoop into the muffin tin and bake for 15 minutes or until a toothpick comes out clean. Set aside for a minute or two and transfer to a wire rack to cool completely.

Baked Apples

Serves 4-5

Prep time: 15 min

Ingredients:

5-6 large apples, peeled

1/2 cup walnuts, crushed

1/3 cup sugar

2 tbsp raisins, soaked

1 tbsp chia seeds

1 tsp vanilla extract

1/2 tsp cinnamon

3 oz butter

Directions:

Carefully hollow out the apple core 3/4 down. Prepare stuffing by combining the butter with sugar, walnuts, raisins, chia seeds, and cinnamon.

Stuff the apples with this mixture and arrange them on an oiled baking dish. Bake for 5-10 minutes at 350 F. Serve warm.

How To Lose Weight (During and) After Menopause?

During the menopause and after it, preventing weight gain is important. Now, more than ever, we need to minimize the intake of empty calories, especially from high-fat, high-sugar foods and we need to stay active. Because, while we can't stop the clock, by exercising and eating right, we can make a real difference to how we feel – and we can stay healthy during and after the menopause and enjoy life more.

Here are some of the easiest things we all can do to maintain a stable and healthy weight.

- Eat a predominantly plant-based diet with lots of protein, good fats, and dietary fiber.
- Eat plenty of fresh fruit that are rich in potassium to help minimize fluid retention.
- Eat little and often to maintain blood sugar levels stable. Instead of sugary snacks and beverages learn to have nuts, seeds and fruit as snacks and water and herbal teas as drinks.
- Make exercise a habit. Find the sports and activities you really like and try to practise at least two times a week. Whenever possible, walk instead of driving.
- Drink plenty of water to ensure good hydration and help maintain body temperature and fluid balance.
- Limit or moderate your intake of salt, as too much salt can affect blood pressure and water retention.
- Keep a positive attitude. Get emotional support from your friends and family.
- Learn to relax: take 30 minutes each day to do something that makes you happy.

FREE BONUS RECIPES: 20 Superfood Paleo and Vegan Smoothies for Vibrant Health and Easy Weight Loss

Kale and Kiwi Smoothie

Serves: 2

Prep time: 2-3 min

Ingredients:

2-3 ice cubes

1 cup orange juice

1 small pear, peeled and chopped

2 kiwi, peeled and chopped

2-3 kale leaves

2-3 dates, pitted

Directions:

Combine all ingredients in a high speed blender and blend until smooth.

Delicious Broccoli Smoothie

Serves: 2

Prep time: 2-3 min

Ingredients:

2-3 frozen broccoli florets

1 cup coconut milk

1 banana, peeled and chopped

1 cup pineapple, cut

1 peach, chopped

1 tsp cinnamon

Directions:

Combine all ingredients in a high speed blender and blend until smooth.

Papaya Smoothie

Serves: 2

Prep time: 2-3 min

Ingredients:

2-3 frozen broccoli florets

1 cup orange juice

1 small ripe avocado, peeled, cored and diced

1 cup papaya

1 cup fresh strawberries

Directions:

Combine all ingredients in a high speed blender and blend until smooth.

Beet and Papaya Smoothie

Serves: 2

Prep time: 2-3 min

Ingredients:

3-4 ice cubes

1 cup orange juice

1 banana, peeled and chopped

1 cup papaya

1 small beet, peeled and cut

Directions:

Combine all ingredients in a high speed blender and blend until smooth.

Lean Green Smoothie

Serves: 2

Prep time: 2-3 min

Ingredients:

1 frozen banana, chopped

1 cup orange juice

2-3 kale leaves, stems removed

1 small cucumber, peeled and chopped

1/2 cup fresh parsley leaves

½ tsp grated ginger

Directions:

Combine all ingredients in a high speed blender and blend until smooth.

Easy Antioxidant Smoothie

Serves: 2

Prep time: 2-3 min

Ingredients:

2-3 frozen broccoli florets

1 cup orange juice

2 plums, cut

1 cup raspberries

1 tsp ginger powder

Directions:

Combine all ingredients in a high speed blender and blend until smooth.

Healthy Purple Smoothie

Serves: 2

Prep time: 2-3 min

Ingredients:

2-3 frozen broccoli florets

1 cup water

1/2 avocado, peeled and chopped

3 plums, chopped

1 cup blueberries

Directions:

Combine all ingredients in a high speed blender and blend until smooth.

Mom's Favorite Kale Smoothie

Serves: 2

Prep time: 2-3 min

Ingredients:

2-3 ice cubes

1½ cup orange juice

1 green small apple, cut

½ cucumber, chopped

2-3 leaves kale

½ cup raspberries

Directions:

Combine all ingredients in a high speed blender and blend until smooth.

Creamy Green Smoothie

Serves: 2

Prep time: 2-3 min

Ingredients:

1 frozen banana

1 cup coconut milk

1 small pear, chopped

1 cup baby spinach

1 cup grapes

1 tbsp coconut butter

1 tsp vanilla extract

Directions:

Combine all ingredients in a high speed blender and blend until smooth.

Strawberry and Arugula Smoothie

Serves: 2

Prep time: 2-3 min

Ingredients:

2 cups frozen strawberries

1 cup unsweetened almond milk

10-12 arugula leaves

1/2 tsp ground cinnamon

Directions:

Combine ice, almond milk, strawberries, arugula and cinnamon in a high speed blender. Blend until smooth and serve.

Emma's Amazing Smoothie

Serves: 2

Prep time: 2-3 min

Ingredients:

1 frozen banana, chopped

1 cup orange juice

1 large nectarine, sliced

1/2 zucchini, peeled and chopped

2-3 dates, pitted

Directions:

Combine all ingredients in a high speed blender and blend until smooth.

Good-To-Go Morning Smoothie

Serves: 2

Prep time: 2-3 min

Ingredients:

1 cup frozen strawberries

1 cup apple juice

1 banana, chopped

1 cup raw asparagus, chopped

1 tbsp ground flaxseed

Directions:

Combine all ingredients in a high speed blender and blend until smooth.

Endless Energy Smoothie

Serves: 2

Prep time: 2-3 min

Ingredients:

1 frozen banana, chopped

1 1/2 cup green tea

1 cup chopped pineapple

2 raw asparagus spears, chopped

1 lime, juiced

1 tbsp chia seeds

Directions:

Combine all ingredients in a high speed blender and blend until smooth.

High-fibre Fruit Smoothie

Serves: 2

Prep time: 2-3 min

Ingredients:

1 frozen banana, chopped

1 cup orange juice

2 cups chopped papaya

1 cup shredded cabbage

1 tbsp chia seeds

Directions:

Combine all ingredients in a high speed blender and blend until smooth.

Nutritious Green Smoothie

Serves: 2

Prep time: 2-3 min

Ingredients:

2-3 frozen broccoli florets

1 cup apple juice

1 large pear, chopped

1 kiwi, peeled and chopped

1 cup spinach leaves

1-2 dates, pitted

Directions:

Combine all ingredients in a high speed blender and blend until smooth.

Apricot, Strawberry and Banana Smoothie

Serves: 2

Prep time: 2-3 min

Ingredients:

1 frozen banana

1 1/2 cup almond milk

5 dried apricots

1 cup fresh strawberries

Directions:

Combine all ingredients in a high speed blender and blend until smooth.

Spinach and Green Apple Smoothie

Serves: 2

Prep time: 2-3 min

Ingredients:

3-4 ice cubes

1 cup unsweetened almond milk

1 banana, peeled and chopped

2 green apples, peeled and chopped

1 cup raw spinach leaves

3-4 dates, pitted

1 tsp grated ginger

Directions:

Combine all ingredients in a high speed blender and blend until smooth.

Superfood Blueberry Smoothie

Serves: 2

Prep time: 2-3 min

Ingredients:

2-3 cubes frozen spinach

1 cup green tea

1 banana

2 cups blueberries

1 tbsp ground flaxseed

Directions:

Combine all ingredients in a high speed blender and blend until smooth.

Zucchini and Blueberry Smoothie

Serves: 2

Prep time: 2-3 min

Ingredients:

1 cup frozen blueberries

1 cup unsweetened almond milk

1 banana

1 zucchini, peeled and chopped

Directions:

Combine all ingredients in a high speed blender and blend until smooth.

Tropical Spinach Smoothie

Serves: 2

Prep time: 2-3 min

Ingredients:

1/2 cup crushed ice or 3-4 ice cubes

1 cup coconut milk

1 mango, peeled and diced

1 cup fresh spinach leaves

4-5 dates, pitted

1/2 tsp vanilla extract

Directions:

Combine all ingredients in a high speed blender and blend until smooth.

About the Author

Alissa Grey is a fitness and nutrition enthusiast who loves to teach people about losing weight and feeling better about themselves. She lives in a small French village in the foothills of a beautiful mountain range with her husband, three teenage kids, two free spirited dogs, and various other animals.

Alissa Grey is incredibly lucky to be able to cook and eat natural foods, mostly grown nearby, something she's done since she was a teenager. She enjoys yoga, running, reading, hanging out with

her family, and growing organic vegetables and herbs.

Made in the USA
Middletown, DE
03 April 2018